Dr. Earl Mindell's

What You Should Know About Homeopathic Remedies

Dr. Earl Mindell's

What You Should Know About Homeopathic Remedies

Earl L. Mindell, R.Ph., Ph.D.

with Virginia L. Hopkins

Keats Publishing, Inc. New Canaan, Connecticut

Dr. Earl Mindell's What You Should Know About Homeopathic Remedies is intended solely for informational and educational purposes, and not as medical advice. Please consult a medical or health professional if you have questions about your health.

DR. EARL MINDELL'S WHAT YOU SHOULD KNOW ABOUT HOMEOPATHIC REMEDIES

Copyright © 1996 by Earl L. Mindell, R.Ph., Ph.D.

Library of Congress Cataloging-in-Publication Data

   [What you should know about homeopathic remedies]
   Dr. Earl Mindell's what you should know about homeopathic remedies / by Earl Mindell and Virginia L. Hopkins.
     p.   cm.
   Includes bibliographical references and index.
   ISBN 0-87983-751-9
   1. Homeopathy—Popular works.   I. Hopkins, Virginia.
RX76.M66   1938
615.5'32—dc20
                                      96-30649
                                          CIP

Printed in the United States of America

Keats Publishing, Inc.
27 Pine Street (Box 876)
New Canaan, Connecticut 06840-0876

98 97 96   6 5 4 3 2 1

CONTENTS

INTRODUCTION

Homeopathy is a healing art that I am not an expert in, but since it is such an effective and safe part of natural healing, I'm including this basic guide to homeopathy in the "What You Should Know" series. Used according to its principles, homeopathy is a powerful tool for healing, especially when used in consultation with an experienced homeopath.

I consider this book a guide to nonserious conditions. If you have a condition such as diabetes, heart disease or severe arthritis, I strongly recommend that you work with an experienced homeopathic practitioner who can offer you the full benefit of these powerful remedies.

Some homeopathic remedies work very quickly and noticeably. For example, with some types of flu, the flu remedy Oscillococcinum can cure symptoms in a matter of hours. Arnica used promptly on a bruise can keep bruising symptoms to a minimum. But if it has taken you a long time to get an illness, a homeopathic remedy is most likely going to take some time, from a few weeks to a few months, to have its effect.

Like all truly effective forms of alternative medicine, homeopathy takes the whole person into account, including the physical, emotional, mental and spiritual levels. It is a form of medicine best used, most of the time, with attention to its principles and with awareness of all the detail that it is capable of addressing. As you delve into homeopathy, and learn to apply its remedies to yourself, you will learn more about an entirely new dimension of yourself, in fascinating detail. When you or your homeopath come upon the correct remedy, you will be amazed at how accurately the list of symptoms for that remedy fits your specific problem.

This guide was written with the assistance of homeopathic practitioner, teacher and author David Dancu, and I recommend that if you want to learn more about homeopathy you take advantage of his book, listed in the reference section in the back of this book, as well as the other works listed. And as I said above, I also recommend that when working with serious conditions, you work with a homeopathic practitioner who can give you the full advantage of the powerful homeopathic remedies.

CHAPTER 1

The History, Science and Philosophy of Homeopathy

Homeopathy originated in the 19th century as a result of the work of a German doctor, Samuel Hahnemann. It is founded on some very specific principles and an extensive list of tested remedies. The remedies are based on natural substances found to have various effects when taken in medicinal doses. The success of homeopathy as a safe and effective form of healing led to growth in its popularity and use throughout the century. As a practice, it was only overtaken when the developing science of modern medicine came to be favored by the medical establishments of North America and Europe.

Almost a century later, the drawbacks and dangers associated with conventional medicine have become obvious. Tranquilizer addiction, birth defects from pregnancy medications, and side effects of common medicines like aspirin, are a few examples of issues which have exposed a darker side to standard medical treatments. Many patients and doctors alike have been prompted to try approaches of a more consistently safe and compassionate nature such as homeopathy.

The tide has turned again in favor of the ancient tradition of medicine which sees the physician in service to the natural power of the body to heal itself. The trend in 20th-century medicine has been toward control and dominance of physical systems in isolation, treating symptoms and pain over and above underlying conditions and causes. Valuable knowledge and techniques have resulted, but often at great cost to the long term health of patients. The aim now is to combine modern developments with the understanding and usefulness of older, proven practices, including homeopathy.

THE LAW OF SIMILARS

Has anyone ever recommended that you "swallow a hair of the dog that bit you?" As a hangover cure it leaves a lot to be desired, but the idea of treating symptoms with a little of a substance that causes them is actually very sound. Known as the "Law of Similars," the theory is ancient. It was part of the writings of philosophers and physicians from Hippocrates to St. Augustine. Herbalists long ago applied a primitive version of the Law of Similars, in the form of the "The Doctrine of Signatures." Some plants were selected for medicinal use because they resembled in some way the part of the body to be treated. The speckled surface of a lungwort leaf, for instance, looks like a lung. Sure enough, modern science shows that the silica in lungwort restores elasticity to lungs and extracts of the plant are useful for reducing bronchial mucus.

A more refined concept of "similarity" was proposed in the 1790s by Samuel Hahnemann.

Unhappy with the increase of the barbaric medical practices of his time such as bloodletting, cupping and mercury poisoning, Hahnemann had quit his medical practice. When he turned to the translation of foreign medical and herbal publications, he began to question their theories and observations, and apply them to his own knowledge of healing.

Folk medicine from South America had produced a treatment for malaria, the world's number one killer disease of the 17th century. Powdered bark from the pretty cinchona tree proved a potent remedy. Known as quinine, cinchona extract is finding favor again today as malarial parasites have become resistant to synthetic drugs. In Hahnemann's time, herbalists believed cinchona's effectiveness was due to its bitterness. Hahnemann was not satisfied with this explanation, since many other bitter herbs were of no help.

Deciding to test the Law of Similars, he dosed himself with extract of cinchona bark. Remarkably, the healthy doctor was inflicted for a short time with symptoms very like those of malaria. This was the first of what Hahnemann called "provings." He continued with the help of colleagues, family and friends to conduct further tests on different substances, keeping detailed records of the results. The provings added further evidence that a cure of symptoms could result from taking herbs, minerals, elements or certain known toxins which actually induced similar responses in healthy people. To summarize his theory, Dr. Hahnemann coined the word "homeopathy" from the Greek words "homoios" for similar and "pathos" for suffering.

HAHNEMANN'S ORGANON AND MATERIA MEDICA

Hahnemann's first book on homeopathy, *The Organon of Rational Medical Science*, was published in 1810. The Organon set out the ideas and philosophy of homeopathy, and Hahnemann explained his systematic approach and theories. These were developed scientifically from the standpoint of someone with a medical degree who was also an authority on metal poisoning and toxicology.

The powerful effects observed by Hahnemann in provings were achieved using highly diluted amounts of the substances involved which, in a few cases, were known poisons. The diluted agents became homeopathic remedies. Over 400 of them were fully described, complete with provings, in his own materia medica, or medical textbook.

Hahnemann's teachings spread slowly throughout Germany, meeting opposition from the entrenched medical establishment. His work was regarded as a threat to much of the German medical world, since he advocated small and limited doses which would not generate large pharmaceutical or practice profits. Personality played a role, too, as Hahnemann's blunt, undiplomatic style won him few friends in established circles.

In spite of the opposition, Hahnemann expanded his writings, refining and adding remedies which led to four further editions of the *Organon* during his lifetime. Through his work with patients, he amassed an additional four volumes of information and cures compiled from cases and patient notes. A sixth *Organon* manuscript lay unpublished until it was found in 1920. This was more than 75 years after Hahnemann's death at age 88, in 1843, some time before homeopathy reached its 19th-century height. The changes and additions to homeopathic theory contained in the sixth *Organon* are major, yet not widely used by many modern homeopaths. The successful results achieved using the first five editions have created a reluctance to change.

THE PHILOSOPHY OF HOMEOPATHY

Even before publication of the *Organon*, Hahnemann's published writings demonstrated a refinement and philosophy that contrasted sharply with the crude thinking behind the common medical practices of the day. Unlike most physicians, he stressed the importance of exercise, diet and hygiene. He was aware of the pioneering work of contemporaries such as Edward Jenner on the smallpox vaccine, and was eager to advance the techniques of the ordinary physician.

Hahnemann's 1796 summary of three main approaches to medical treatment remains valid today. The first type of treatment could remove a known cause of a disease. A second form worked to oppose the effects of a disease, such as antacids to relieve heartburn, for example. The third, and superior type in his view, was treatment with similars designed to support the self-healing capabilities of the body. This was the essence of homeopathy. Hahnemann regarded homeopathic treatment, and prevention, as the only truly valid approaches to medicine. Each leads to the maintenance or active restoration of health rather than to the removal or suppression of disease factors.

Hahnemann understood the role of disease agents, but emphasized the idea that each person has a predisposition, or tendency, to get certain types of illness. He observed that agents act as triggers for disease, but not in all cases, and with worse consequences for some people than others. For example, the flu may afflict half the people in the office, and the other half may be unaffected. This led him to argue that the condition of the person is of greater importance than the disease agent. Included in this concept was the idea of the *vital force* of the individual, a term used by Hahnemann to explain the constant, automatic drive of an organism to stay in a healthy state.

HOMEOPATHY IN THE 19TH CENTURY

An increasing number of followers led to the rapid spread of homeopathy to almost all European countries as well as the United States, Mexico, Cuba and Russia. Eventually it would also reach South America and India. One of the main reasons for the growth in homeopathy was its superior effect in the treatment of epidemics such as typhoid fever and cholera which swept over Europe and America in the last century. When yellow fever hit the southern states of America in 1878, death rates were one third fewer in patients treated with homeopathy than in those receiving orthodox treatment. In London, in 1854, over half the cholera patients in conventional hospitals died, in contrast to just over 16 percent in homeopathic hospitals.

Homeopathy was introduced to the United States in 1825. Demand for homeopathy in America stemmed initially from German communities. Philadelphia saw the establishment of the first homeopathic medical school in 1833. The school was founded by Dr. Constantine Hering who had originally taken up the cause against Hahnemann in Germany. Aimed at disproving the discoveries of homeopathy, Hering's research did the opposite! Convinced by a natural form of healing free of side effects, the former enemy became a dedicated ally. Hering went on to write many books on homeopathy and himself worked as a homeopathic practitioner.

Another famous American homeopath was James Kent, M.D. who was based in Philadelphia from the early 1890s. Many years of work, involving the treatment of over 30,000 patients, and lectures and notes from other materia medica, led to the publication in 1897 of *Kent's Repertory*. As a comprehensive listing of symptoms and remedies, this source is still used by homeopaths everywhere.

Leading proponents such as Hering and Kent worked to meet the rising call for homeopathy in America which, by the 1880s, had created 100 hospitals and 20 medical colleges. Homeopathy was taught at Boston, Iowa, Michigan and Minnesota universities. At that time, twenty percent of physicians were homeopaths. The gentle approach of homeopathy, free of side effects, and caring for the patient as a whole, was in contrast to the rising use of synthetic drugs and treatment only of symptoms in standard American medical practice.

PRESSURES AGAINST HOMEOPATHY

Patients in the 18th century were accustomed to brutal techniques like mercury dosing, which frequently caused teeth to fall out, and bloodletting often "until four fifths of the blood contained in the body are drawn away!" Homeopathy provided an attractive alternative. Ordinary folk and the elite of society, including politicians and the wealthy, patronized homeopaths, competing with standard physicians. The resulting jealousy and fear meant homeopathy became the target of official repression. The founding of the American Institute of Homeopathy in 1844 was followed, as a direct response, two years later by the formation of the American Medical Association (AMA). Doctors with any connections to homeopathic practices were barred from the AMA. Members of the AMA were not even permitted to consult homeopaths.

The pharmaceutical industry also perceived itself threatened by homeopathy. Scientists in the 18th century had discovered that the active chemicals of medicinal plants could be isolated. During the 19th century, chemists focused on the extraction and synthesis of these potent substances. In the minds of industry and public alike was the idea of quick-fix, one-stop medicine. Long term effects and treatment of underlying conditions came to be largely ignored. New, synthesized drugs were often speedily effective against urgent symptoms. Side effects went unidentified as drugs could treat those, too, masking true medicinal changes in the body.

Additional pressure came when the United States government commissioned the Flexner Report in 1910. The intention was to assess medical education and to set standard practices. However, this was in the context of the rise of a limited chemical approach fixated on physical symptoms. The report led to the closure of many medical schools, including those teaching homeopathy. Homeopathy fell outside the narrow biochemical framework accepted and promoted by the medical establishment. It has to be added that homeopaths created their own vulnerability to attack. As a developing system, it accommodated proponents of different views on high and low dilutions and did not offer a consistent front to those attempting to undermine the subject. Millions of dollars' worth of grants were denied to homeopathic medical schools, and homeopathic hospitals became standard medical institutions.

Adding to the decline of homeopathy in the United Sates was a major lifestyle shift from slow-paced and rural to urban and mobile. Society no longer provided an easy fit for the typical family doctor who often treated the same patients for their entire lives. Finally, the advent of so-called "wonder drugs" in the 1940s saw homeopathy retreat outside the margins of medical practice.

HOMEOPATHY TODAY

It wasn't until the early 1970s that dissatisfaction within the medical field led to a revival of homeopathy. Recognizing the ineffectiveness and often downright harm of modern drugs, some physicians arranged to study in Greece where homeopathy was more widely practiced. Greek instructors came to America to lecture on Hahnemann's work, and so began the increase in popularity of homeopathy seen in the United States today.

More than one-third of the U.S. population now uses alternative remedies, including homeopathy. Complications from prescription drugs result in 40 percent of hospitalizations and cause 20,000 to 30,000 deaths every year in the United States. The comparative effectiveness and safety of homeopathic remedies is being demonstrated by more and more top-notch scientific studies done by respected institutes. Studies done in America, England, Germany, Holland and France include research into homeopathic remedies for cold and flu, skin ailments, allergies, insect bites and stings, menopause and sports injuries.

In America, homeopathic remedies are now recognized as medicines. They are freely available in health and drug stores and come under the jurisdiction of the Food and Drug Administration (FDA). Some homeopathic remedies, such as nitroglycerine for certain heart ailments, have been taken up by allopathic medicine and used in medicinal doses.

The Queen of England and Mother Theresa have homeopathy in common! The Queen is attended by a homeopathic physician and homeopathic remedies are used in Mother Theresa's Calcutta hospital. Homeopathic medicines are used in the practices of a fifth of German physicians and just under a third of French physicians.

In 1980, there were nearly 800 homeopathic doctors in France and around 200 in Britain. India boasts about 124 homeopathic medical schools and there is a sprinkling of schools and colleges in South America. About 450 homeopathic physicians practice in Argentina alone.

Aside from entrenched medical practice steered to a large degree by drug company interests, there has remained a mainstream reluctance to accept homeopathy. This has been due in part to the fact that no complete understanding of what makes homeopathy effective exists. Another factor is the lack of interest on the part of homeopaths to finding classifiable, physical causes to the symptoms it cures. Allopathic medicine has yet to move on to the position that the agents of disease are less important than the paths that lead to recovery and cure.

Those practicing homeopathy have begun to realize the need to move on as well, and accept the need for testing that meets the criteria of Western medicine as well as established techniques of proving. Perhaps the time has come for the gentle, proven techniques of homeopathy to gain acceptance alongside the best and safest of current established medical practices.

PUTTING HOMEOPATHY TO THE TEST

Homeopathy is an ongoing subject of research and an interesting one because the way it works is not completely understood, although there are some very convincing theories. Impartial and well executed studies include work on a range of subjects. In an article in the *British Medical Journal*,

107 controlled trials in homeopathy were reviewed by authors who were not themselves homeopaths. Most of the trials did not meet Western medicine protocals, but nevertheless, the authors were amazed at the amount of positive evidence that could still be gleaned. Many more trials are needed to satisfy scientific criteria, but headway is already being made.

Examples of recent homeopathic trials include a Harvard clinical study on Similasan Eye Drops # 2, an ophthalmic (eye) allergy medication containing extracts of honey bee, eyebright and cevadilla. Using a well-established test known as the Antigen Challenge, the drops were found to significantly reduce hay fever symptoms such as itching and bloodshot eyes.

According to a study published in the *The Lancet*, a homeopathic remedy was more effective than a placebo in relieving allergy symptoms (mainly due to dust mites) in 28 patients who also continued their conventional care. Patients taking the homeopathic remedy reported 33 percent fewer asthma symptoms, sustained for up to four weeks after the trial. Improvements were seen within one week from the start of the treatment. These results correlated with a 53 percent increase in histamine resistance for the treated group, while the placebo group saw a 7 percent decrease.

In a study of 81 children in Nicaragua, reported in the journal *Pediatrics*, children treated with a homeopathic medicine for diarrhea recovered more quickly than those given a placebo.

A 1995 clinical study of 68 volunteers, published in the *European Journal of Clinical Pharmacol-*

ogy, found a homeopathic gel to be significantly superior to a placebo in the treatment of mosquito bites.

Results such as these give a hint of the wide-ranging use and effectiveness of homeopathic medicines. It should be noted, too, that this is without the application of full homeopathic techniques, which require exact tailoring of remedies to the individual affected, not just the physical symptoms in isolation.

THE PRINCIPLES OF HOMEOPATHY

A basic, guiding principle of homeopathy was stated by Hahnemann in his *Organon*: "The highest ideal of therapy is to restore health rapidly, gently, permanently; to remove and destroy the whole disease in the shortest, surest, least harmful way, according to clearly comprehensible principles."

Hahnemann developed just such specific principles which are still followed, shaping the practice of all homeopaths today.

The Principle of The Like Remedy

A homeopathic remedy always follows the Law of Similars, as it is chosen for its ability to produce symptoms that are most like those of the person to be treated. For instance, the syrup of ipecacuanha will cause vomiting when ingested in its natural form. When diluted and potentized in the homeopathic form (this concept will be explained shortly), it prevents or eliminates vomiting and nausea. This is considered the foundation for homeopathic principles; whatever causes a specific reaction in an individual also cures that disharmony when taken in homeopathic dilution.

In homeopathy, symptoms are investigated in depth, covering physical signs, the nature of the illness, underlying level of health and energy, personality, trauma and inherited tendencies. The aim is always to look at the person as a whole. Remedies are chosen from a range that has been scientifically tested on healthy human beings to determine what symptoms they produce. The resulting list of symptoms is known as a remedy's "drug picture." One of the fundamental discoveries of homeopathy showed that the most effective remedy is the one whose drug picture most closely matches the individual's symptoms, or "clinical picture."

The Single Drug Principle

Many combination homeopathic remedies are effective for acute illnesses or conditions. In our fast-paced lives, when there isn't time to stop and review symptoms in depth, a combination remedy often does the trick. However, it will leave you without knowledge as to which homeopathic substance in particular was most effective. Combinations are not original homeopathic remedies, but derive more from the herbalist approach, where long tradition shows that different agents can enhance the effect of others.

Classic homeopathy calls for one remedy to be tried at a time so that its effects can be clearly seen. If unrelated symptoms or symptoms not experienced before should occur after taking a homeopathic dose, the remedy should be discontinued. Any ill effects, however, will be short lived.

The Principle of the Small Dose and Potentization

One fascinating discovery made by Hahnemann was that the effectiveness of a homeopathic remedy increased the more the dose was diluted. Hahnemann observed that when a match was achieved between symptoms and a remedy, the patient would be very sensitive to the remedy. A much lower dose was needed for a positive reaction than in a case without a good symptom match or in a healthy person. This spurred Hahnemann to continue lowering dilutions to find curative doses as well as to eradicate toxicity.

Part of the process of dilution involved vigorous shaking, called succussion, to achieve useable, homogeneous chemical solutions. Hahnemann later named this process *potentization* or *dynamization*. Achieving increased potency with lower doses is in contrast to allopathy, where normally the dose is *increased* to produce more effect.

In his fifth edition of the *Organon*, Hahnemann sets out a range of potencies. The most commonly used dilutions are given in centesimal and decimal amounts. In centesimal potencies, one drop of the active substance is dissolved in 99 drops of distilled water, alcohol or glycerine. Substances which cannot be dissolved in this way are ground up with lactose (milk sugar). A resulting solution is called the mother tincture, which is then used as the basis for further dilution, producing potency ranges termed 1c right up to 100,000c or cm. Decimal, or x potencies, involve dilution of the mother tincture in just 9 drops of water or alcohol. X potencies range from 1x to 200x. Much weaker solutions, known as lm potencies, were recommended by Hahnemann in his sixth *Organon*, but these have not been widely used.

The Principle of the Infrequent Dose

Homeopathic remedies are only administered as necessary. With acute, self-limiting conditions such as bruises and colds, the right remedy can produce changes four to eight hours or even sooner after the first dose. Patience, however, is part of the key to homeopathic treatment of more serious conditions. Days and sometimes weeks are allowed for effects to be seen and doses are not repeated when improvement is maintained. There is no expectation of the long, continuous courses of medicine often seen with allopathic medicine.

The Principle of Noninterference with the Body's Natural Response

This principle recognizes the body's innate ability to heal itself. There is much greater knowledge today than during Hahnemann's time of the numerous repair functions of the body. When struck by illness or injury, the body automatically triggers healing processes on many levels. For example, fevers burn off infections, endorphins flow as natural pain killers, and white blood cells destroy foreign agents. Although the exact nature of the healing systems was not known to Hahnemann, he recognized and summarized these kinds of responses and their regulatory mechanism as vital reactions.

We now know exactly how conventional 19th century medical practices such as bloodletting would have literally drained the body's ability to respond to infection. Hahnemann observed as much, even though he was unaware of the precise processes being crudely ignored. For this reason he formulated the principle of noninterference. Homeopathy is designed to support the healing functions of the body, shortening the time needed to restore health.

The Principle of Treatment of the Whole Person

Hahnemann observed that the body's ability to fight disease and repair itself was directed by what he referred to as the *vital force*. This was his description of the capacity of organisms to self-regulate always in the direction of survival and therefore health. Even today, this function is not well understood, but, like Hahnemann, we see it affected by moods and emotions. Today, we can measure how immune cell numbers drop with depression or how our body's natural anticancer agents increase with happiness. By acknowledging a vital force, Hahnemann was addressing the large role played by the emotional, mental and spiritual levels of a person's health.

A good homeopathic assessment reviews a person's vitality and emotional state. If someone has a cold but still feels energetic, a more potent remedy will be tolerated. Similarly, acute symptoms such as a cold are not treated homeopathically without regard also to chronic conditions such as arthritis or indigestion.

Thorough training in all aspects of homeopathy leads to the most comprehensive and effective treatments. This is why it makes good sense to select a trained, experienced homeopath.

HOW DOES HOMEOPATHY WORK?

The answer to this question is not fully known. The powerful effect of the very diluted remedies used in homeopathy is a puzzling subject for researchers. Many dilutions are so high that no molecular trace of the original substance can be found. Homeopaths believe that the vigorous shaking at each level of dilution leaves the energy of the original dissolved substance imprinted on the medium of solution, something like an energetic blueprint, or fingerprint.

Various theories about the mechanisms of homeopathy are being tested. For example, electromagnetism may play a role, as it has been found that allergic manifestations occur in highly sensitive subjects contacting water treated with electromagnetic frequencies. Some investigations suggest that when pure water is treated with electromagnetic waves it gains new physical and chemical properties that are conserved for some time. It's true to say that the properties of water are in many ways still a mystery. Results of future work investigating homeopathic dilutions may yield interesting discoveries.

Homeopathy can be seen as influencing the energy fields of the body. Each human body is a unique pattern of energy flows and each cell has an electromagnetic or "bioelectric" field. A cell is an energy generator, functioning in harmony with every other cell to create an overall level of health. At times of illness, there are disharmonies in energy production and flows in the body.

It is thought that the properties of a correct homeopathic remedy for an ailment in some way resonate with and strengthen the body's efforts to realign its unbalanced energy flows.

WORKING WITH, NOT AGAINST, SYMPTOMS

When you take a dose of, say, antibiotics, the aim is to kill the organisms that have caused the symptoms of an infection. You might also take other drugs to bring down a fever or kill pain. This, of course, is very different from the approach taken by homeopathy. Allopathic treatment has a vital role in emergency treatment and it gets results because it often removes the source of an infection or condition. However, it usually does so with a blast of powerful substances that override the body's own defense mechanisms. In many cases, allopathic medicine simply suppresses symptoms and does not tackle root causes. This is true, for instance, of drugs for heartburn, sinus troubles and high blood pressure. In addition, the medicinal substances themselves frequently cause unwanted side effects which not uncommonly lead to the administration of yet more drugs.

In homeopathy, symptoms are regarded as outward signs of the body's efforts to repair itself. By taking tiny amounts of a substance which produces similar symptoms, a cure results because the defense work of the body has been stimulated and reinforced. In allopathic medicine, the disease often becomes harder to treat, as with bacteria that become resistant to antibiotics. The aim of homeopathy is not to bypass the body's own systems, but to support them. In this way the body gains in its ability to fend off disease.

Release of Suppressed Symptoms

Hahnemann's provings showed that a remedy can provoke an "occasional initial aggravation," the release of symptoms which have become suppressed. When a release is seen it is sometimes referred to as a healing crisis. A release involves the recurrence of old symptoms, usually for just a few hours a day, but sometimes longer if they were originally severe. A trained homeopathic doctor will decide whether to prescribe a different remedy, reduce the potency, or wait out the crisis.

In allopathic medicine, it is unlikely that a patient would be asked to consider past symptoms. A reappearance of old symptoms may be seen as incidental and/or subject to new treatment, or mistaken as a sign that a successful treatment should be changed. Allopathic medicine is unlikely to consider a recurrence of old symptoms as a sign of recovery.

Disease as a Dynamic Condition

The tendency in allopathic medicine is to fit the patient to a known disease. A doctor attempts to pin down symptoms to a generally classified pattern, in which the overall match is more important than any variations shown by an individual. This is what medical doctors are taught in medical school: first they learn how to diagnose a disease, and then they learn which drug to prescribe to treat the disease. We've all seen doctors prescribe a first choice of antibiotics and then a second, even a third, when the first was ineffective. People have become used to being treated in such a general fashion, since modern medicine has established certain "molds" for illness to fit into. At the same time, we accept that people experience disease differently, recovering at different rates, responding to viruses with different symptoms, requiring more or less rest. Yet despite these observed differences, we've learned to accept nonindividualized treatment.

Homeopathy and the Holistic Approach

Holistic treatment does not single out one physical aspect or body part for treatment. It is an approach that takes the whole person into account, rather than just physical symptoms. As an holistic practice, homeopathy does not place the disease in a compartment separate from the individual. Symptoms are seen to reflect ongoing, dynamic efforts by the body to return to a healthy state, not as unwanted manifestations to be classified and stamped out in isolation from other bodily functions.

In this way, homeopathy recognizes the interdependency of all parts of the body. It also incorporates the role played by personality types so that homeopathic treatments are tuned to each individual patient.

THE HOMEOPATHIC PHYSICIAN

Most physicians are well-intentioned and sincere in their vocation. The training of an allopathic doctor, however, is steered toward acceptance of a prescription drug culture, in which the medical world is greatly influenced by the pharmaceutical industry. The homeopath takes a more independent view, although his or her training in medical matters will be just as thorough. A homeopath perceives his or her prescriptions as supplementary rather than superior to the body's own powers. In practicing homeopathy, a physician will usually pay greater attention to the patient's general condition than an allopathic doctor. A desire to know a great deal about individual patients and their symptoms in great detail leads to much more time spent with them than is the norm in conventional medicine. Whereas a standard physician may see about 30 patients a day, spending about 10 minutes with each, a homeopathic doctor typically sees 8 to10 patients a day and spends about an hour with each one.

Like any other doctor, a homeopathic physician receives an M.D. degree and his or her state license to practice medicine. To qualify to practice homeopathy, he or she then goes on to a postgraduate course in the subject, followed by a period of work with a practicing homcopathic physician. Only a few states license homeopathic practitioners. Recommendations from others and experience count equally for conventional and homeopathic doctors.

What to Expect from a Homeopathic Physician

You may understand how a homeopathic doctor is different from an allopathic physician, but how does this affect treatment? Homeopathy sets out certain procedures as standard. As a result, patients can expect a basic similarity in the work of different homeopaths. As with doctors of all kinds, of course, each physician has his or her own style and character which will influence the way he or she practices.

One of the major preferences expressed by those who choose a homeopathic doctor is over the amount of time the physician is willing to spend with patients. An initial hour-long interview is typical, and feedback from patients is welcome in regard to the changes seen after taking a remedy. Important and specific use is made of patient-doctor time.

A standard element of homeopathy is the collection of information about the patient. This is known as "taking the case." From the first encounter with the patient, a homeopathic doctor is taking note of his or her condition. Factual information is recorded, including age, occupation, marital status and the patient's reason for visiting. A homeopath goes on from there to consider factors such as posture, complexion, stress level, and emotions as valuable clues to an individual's state of health. Considerable skill is needed for a homeopath to be sure of noting underlying traits, not just accept a doctor's-visit façade!

An interview notes not just physical symptoms, their onset, type and timing, but also personal history, which provides information about a patient's emotional and mental tendencies—if they are ambitious, inhibited or extroverted, for example. A history of family illness is also covered, to give an indication of any possible inherited conditions, and the individual's probable underlying physical strengths and weaknesses.

Symptoms are discussed in detail, determining how they have changed and if they vary over the day. In addition, the patient is asked to describe how his or her condition affects him or her, and if it has changed the way they react to their environment. Food preferences are important here, noting, for instance, if something is disliked that was previously favored.

The result of the initial interview is a comprehensive picture of the patient's state of health, specific symptoms, and personal response to their condition. The homeopathic physician uses the interview notes as the basis for prescribing a remedy without the need arising to first classify the illness.

Visiting a physician for a full homeopathic review results in the prescription of a single remedy. This is to avoid stimulating multiple responses in the body which cannot be definitely associated with a specific remedy. In other words, a homeopath's initial intention is to find only the remedy which is key to the illness. This approach is very different from an individual's educated purchase of a combination remedy for self-treatment.

Someone finding quick relief, say, from hay fever, isn't going to mind exactly which substance in a combination remedy produces the result. More severe conditions, however, merit a comprehensive investigation, which leads in traditional homeopathy to one remedy alone.

Diagnosis Comes Second to Symptoms

The pattern of symptoms observed by a homeopathic physician is used to point to a specific remedy rather than to a particular disease. This is called "constitutional prescribing," or matching the treatment to the person as a whole, not just the condition. Homeopaths do provide a diagnosis if one is needed, say, for insurance purposes, but the diagnosis is not used to provide the framework for action.

Out of perhaps a dozen main symptoms, the physician will usually judge five or so to be the strongest. One symptom may point to several remedies. Exactly which remedy is used is determined in cross-reference with the remedies suggested by the other leading symptoms. Usually, one remedy will match most of the symptoms. The physician checks the description of patient and symptoms listed under the remedy to insure it is indeed a clear match with the individual being treated. A good match between the "drug picture" and the "clinical picture" is confirmation that the right remedy has been selected. The remedy is prescribed and any dietary factors, such as coffee, which could interfere with its actions, are ruled out. Most homeopaths provide general advice about diet and lifestyle, since prevention of disease is a high priority in the homeopathic world. The first visit, however, is usually reserved for "taking the case" and dealing with immediate discomfort.

AGGRAVATION AS A COMMON RESPONSE

The old adage "you'll feel worse before you feel better" often holds truth in homeopathy. A patient is usually very sensitive to the right remedy, which produces symptoms most similar to his own. The right remedy will often provoke the defensive measures of the body, and often actually increases the intensity of symptoms for as long as a day or two. This syndrome of aggravation can also be the release of earlier, repressed symptoms.

An expert homeopath will be sure to confirm that any increase in symptoms is either a temporary, bearable worsening of symptoms or a renewal of old ones, rather than a new set of responses which are not connected to the original condition being treated.

KEEPING COSTS DOWN

One bonus of homeopathic treatment is that it is less costly than allopathic medicine. Visits are made less frequently and fewer diagnostic tests are ordered. A century and a half of research, provings and contributions to materia medica means that homeopathic pharmaceutical companies do not have to bear the huge costs of research and development of new drugs. A homeopathic physician prescribes from an established range of about 500 classically proven homeopathic substances, and a total of about 2,800 substances, which are produced without expensive hype and promotion. The result is medications for prescription and self-treatment which are cheaper than the conventional medicines. An allopathic doctor, in contrast, has a prescription list of about 10,000 available drugs whose high cost reflects the high price of their manufacture and promotion.

Homeopathic drugs are safe. The long history of their production and use has insured they are nontoxic. Modern medical drugs, on the other hand, lead to an estimated five to 10 million serious reactions every year. The costs of treating adverse drug reactions does not arise with homeopathy.

THE PATIENT'S ROLE

Anyone seeking homeopathic treatment benefits from a willingness to be honest and thorough in communication with the physician. A homeopathic patient-doctor relationship is a close and active one. The patient is not a passive recipient of advice and treatment. Finding an effective homeopathic remedy relies on good communication from a patient willing to convey a lot of information about his condition. With a remedy in use, the patient's job is to provide feedback about any and all changes. Strong communication creates a close and effective relationship between homeopathic patient and doctor. This helps the doctor ensure the appropriate medicine is in use and that no condition needing allopathic intervention has been missed. Unlike allopathic patients, who are expected to quietly and passively do as they are told without question, homeopathic patients are expected to speak up loud and clear!

CHAPTER 2

Self-Treating and Using Combination Remedies and Formulas

Combination remedies have been used in homeopathy since its beginnings. One of Samuel Hahnemann's first combinations, Causticum, was a mixture of slaked lime with a solution of potassium sulphate. Its effectiveness was clear and powerful. This unique combination remedy covers many conditions, including joint problems, emotional disharmonies, allergies, fibromyalgia, sinus problems, back pains, and multiple sclerosis.

There are several things to consider when choosing either a combination remedy or a combination of remedies. Most classical homeopaths use only single remedies, simply because they can determine the effect of that remedy without interaction of other forces. With each single remedy, there is a clear proving of what that remedy can cause.

Simplicity is the underlying key for using homeopathy, and single remedies provide the basis for maintaining that simplicity. Combinations, on the other hand, are easy to use for self-treatment, but may not be as effective for chronic conditions, such as asthma, arthritis, depression, anxiety or most other long-term illnesses.

Let's say I have been getting headaches frequently. They usually occur after stress or possibly from a reaction to car exhaust. There are three approaches to consider. The obvious and easy one is the traditional western philosophy of taking an aspirin to eliminate the headache. The second approach is to try a homeopathic combination containing five or six remedies, all generally specific for headaches, such as Nux Vomica, Spigilia, Sanguinaria or Lycopodium. One of these will probably work just fine, much like an aspirin.

The third approach, which is a more classical homeopathic approach, uses a different perspective, as it considers the cause of the headache, not just the symptom. One remedy is given based on the whole picture, rarely just the headache alone. This way, a determination is made on both the effect and the result, while also considering whether or not there were reactions in other parts of the body.

The first two approaches look to the symptom without consideration for the person or the cause. And there are obvious times when this approach is not only effective but necessary. Whenever possible though, a review of all symptoms will help to establish a deeper, more permanent healing.

In addition to having specific labels for various ailments, ranging from colds to asthma, combination remedies list a series of ingredients. Reputable companies make these combinations, based on sound homeopathic principles. They combine remedies which work for the ailment described on the label, specifically derived from established materia medica (a book describing remedies) and provings.

Each homeopathic remedy chosen is based on clear symptoms of mental, emotional and physical aspects. A good example is a remedy called pulsatilla. Emotionally, the symptom picture of this remedy is generally a codependent, weepy, timid, depressed, capricious and soft woman. Physically, she often has PMS, stomach or digestive disorders, hay fever, headaches, joint problems and is rarely thirsty, despite a dry mouth.

Typically she is also warm-blooded, with most of her symptoms being much worse either in the sun or in a stuffy, warm room. Her skin is frequently fair, she has light-colored hair and is overweight. Visualize a vine, clinging to the side of a building, and you have a good picture of Pulsatilla tendencies. A healthy person taking this remedy may exhibit some of the above symptoms. But this also demonstrates what it can cure when taken by someone who has similar symptoms.

Every proven homeopathic remedy has its own unique portrait, some in more depth than others. And some are more specific to certain ailments, such as berberis for kidney and bladder problems. The number of proven remedies is about 2,800, with more added on a regular basis.

There are also quite a few substances being called homeopathic that have never been proven and have no relationship to cure other than the fact that they have been diluted. It takes time and effort to weed out the proven from the unproven, but the time taken may prevent ill effects or an unwanted proving on yourself.

All proven remedies are listed in a book called a materia medica. It gives necessary information and effects of each specific remedy. Ask your health food store to carry an inexpensive version for review purposes. You can also use this book and the others recommended in the back of the book for proven recommendations.

Remedies that are proven combinations often naturally occur that way. This list includes calcium and phosphorus, iron and phosphorus, sodium and sulphur and hundreds of others. The idea is to understand what the combination may create and what effect it will have on the body, once created.

For an acute problem or an emergency, combinations can be very helpful and effective. In chronic or long-term disharmonies, the combination remedies act much in the same way as an aspirin does, rarely getting to the cause, just giving temporary relief. And continued repetition is necessary to maintain that relief.

The following is a review of specific remedies in relation to general areas of the body. When considering a combination for a certain ailment, one or more of these remedies would generally be included. Keep in mind that each remedy may be valuable for more than one type of illness or ailment. For instance, Arsenicum Album is a single remedy used for allergies, sneezing, diarrhea, colitis, skin problems, respiratory ailments, shingles, headaches, food poisoning, fears, anxieties, compulsive disorders and depression. But it is best used when there is restlessness in conjunction with one of the above ailments, because otherwise it may not be as effective or long lasting.

The headings described below, along with related remedies, should be used as guidelines, rather than absolutes. Remember that some substances being called homeopathic remedies have never been proven, and unless one of the listed remedies is included, use caution in your selections.

The Head (including headache, injury, pains and congestion): Arnica; Aconite; Belladonna; China; Gelsemium; Glonine; Iris; Kali Bichromium; Lachesis; Natrum Muriaticum; Nux Vomica; Phosphorus; Pulsatilla; Sepia; Silica; Sulphur.

The Nose (including sinus, pains, congestion and discharges): Aconite; Allium Cepa; Arsenicum Iodatum; Belladonna; Calcarea Carbonica; Euphrasia; Hepar; Kali Bichromium; Lycopodium; Mercurius; Natrum Muriaticum; Pulsatilla; Silica; Sticta; Thuja.

The Mouth (including abscesses, odor, pains and infections): Arsenicum Album; Calcarea Carbonica and Phosphoricum; Camphora; China; Carbo Vegetabilisatablis; Hepar; Mercurius; Nitricum Acidum; Lachesis; Nux Vomica; Silica; Sulphur.

The Eyes (including injuries, vision, eruptions, discharges, inflammations, pains and styes): Apis; Aconite; Euphrasia; Ruta; Staphysagria; Causticum; Phosphorus; Pulsatilla; Natrum Muriaticum; Nitricum Acidum; Mercurius; Kreosotum; Rhus Tox; Silica.

The Ears (including infections, hearing, pains and tinnitus): Aconite; Belladonna; Chamomilla; Pulsatilla; Silica; Hepar Sulphuricum; Mercurius; Kali Bichromium; Sulphur; Causticum; Petroleum; Lycopodium; Sarsaparilla; China.

The Throat (including infection, inflammation and pains): Aconite; Apis; Arsenicum Album; Belladonna; Cantharis; Phytolacca; Sulphur; Phosphorus; Pulsatilla; Lycopodium; Mercurius; Lachesis; Natrum Muriaticum; Rhus Tox; Silica; Capsicum.

The Lungs (including inflammations, infections, breathing, coughs and discharges): Arsenicum Album; Antimonium Tart; Argentum Nitricum; Bryonia; Carcinosin; Drosera; Hepar; Kali Bichromium; Lachesis; Phosphorus; Rumex Tuberculinum; Spongia; Sambucus; Sulphur.

The Stomach (including digestion, gas, bloating, pains, cramps, appetite, hiccoughs and nausea): Antimonium Crudum; Argentum Nitricum; Arsenicum Album; Carbo Vegetabilisatablis; Calcarea Carbonica; China; Chelidonium; Ipecacuanha; Cocculus Indicus; Lachesis; Lycopodium; Nux Vomica; Aloe; Natrum Muriaticum; Pulsatilla.

Extremities (including joints, pains, bones, bruises, breaks, arthritis, inflammations, ligaments and strains): Arnica; Calcarea Carbonica; Calcarea Fluorica; Calcarea Phosphorica; Causticum; Colchicum; Cuprum; Silica; Symphytum;

Phosphorus; Plumbum; Bryonia; Rhus Tox Ruta; Ledum.

Female (including PMS, hormonal problems, cysts, herpes, pains, menopause, discharges and headaches): Belladonna; Calcarea Carbonica; Caulophyllum; Cimicifuga; Cyclamen; Ignacia; Lilium Tig; Natrum Muriaticum; Natrum Carbonicum; Natrum Phosphoricum; Phosphorus; Sepia; Pulsatilla; Platina; Sabina; Lycopodium; Thuja; Silica; Kreosotum; Medorrhinum; Nitricum Acidum.

Male (including herpes, impotence, erectile difficulty, prostate, pains, desires, infections and inflammations): Arsenicum Album; Argentum Nitricum; Calcarea Carbonica; Calcarea Sulphuricum; Causticum; Conium; Lycopodium; Nux Vomica; Medorrhinum; Lachesis; Thuja; Sabal; Sulphur; Mercurius.

Sleep (including insomnia, thoughts, disturbed, restless, anxious; too short or too long and unrefreshing): Arsenicum Album; Argentum Nitricum; Belladonna; Calcarea Carbonica; Causticum; Chamomilla; China; Carcinosin; Coffea; Lachesis; Lycopodium; Nux Vomica; Rhus Tox; Phosphorus; Pulsatilla; Thuja; Sulphur; Silica; Ignacia; Natrum Muriaticum.

Fevers (including infections, inflammation, viral, bacterial, malarial and nervous): Aconite; Arsenicum Album; Baptisia; Belladonna; China; Bryonia; Gelsemium; Hepar Sulphuricum; Lycopodium; Natrum Muriaticum; Nux Vomica; Phosphorus; Pyrogenium; Rhus Tox; Silica; Stramonium; Sulphur.

Organs (including liver, spleen, heart, kidney, bladder, brain and gallbladder): Arsenicum Album; Apis; Cantharis; Calcarea Carbonica; China; Ceanothus; Cardus Marianus; Alumina; Crataegus; Aurum; Berberis; Equisetum; Cheledonium; Lycopodium; Lachesis; Natrum Mur; Phosphorus; Nux Vomica; Belladonna.

The Mind (including anxiety, fears, confidence, anger, despair, confusion, blame, mental exhaustion, grief, guilt, mental restlessness, apathy, impatience, sensitive, stubborn, shy, suicidal and worried): Aconite; Aurum; Arsenicum Album; Argentum Nitricum; Causticum; Calcarea Carbonica; Calcarea Phosphoricum; Carcinosin; Kali Carbonicum; Ignacia; Lycopodium; Nux Vomica; Natrum Muriaticum; Natrum Phosphoricum; Mercurius; Nitricum Acidum; Phosphoric Acidum; Phosphorus; Stramonium; Silica; Sulphur; Thuja.

As mentioned earlier, there are over 2,800 proven remedies, and it would be impossible to include all of the appropriate ones in the headings just described. But, generally speaking, you will find that one or more of the remedies mentioned above are frequently included in a combination.

The main reason to take a formula or combination remedy is to get well or recover from an illness or accident. This recovery should be quick, painless and without side effects. Just as important for some is the low cost of the remedies in comparison to typical medical expenditures.

Using formula remedies essentially covers each

of these components, especially in acute or short-acting ailments. The remedy best suited to the illness is often found within the combination, as there may be up to 10 remedies combined in a formula. In effect, it is just the one that fits the disharmony that helps to alleviate it, while the others are rendered inert by the very effectiveness of the productive one.

An example of someone with allergies can demonstrate how this works. A 24-year-old woman has allergies to ragweed with the following symptoms: sneezing; burning, tearing eyes; itching throat; runny nose with a clear, watery discharge; head feels stuffy or congested; occasional wheezing with cough.

Combination remedies for allergies would generally include: Allium Cepa; Arsenicum Album; Euphrasia; Arundo; Wyethia; Sabadilla; Ambrosia; and possibly Nux Vomica, Arsenicum Iodatum or Natrum Muriaticum. There is one remedy that stands out above all the others and fits each of the allergic symptoms described in the example above, Ambrosia.

As Ambrosia so closely matches these symptoms, it eliminates them, brings about balance in the body and more or less negates the other listed remedies. Allergies disappear, the immune system becomes stronger and after a few more doses, the symptoms may not even return. All because the best suited remedy fit the symptom picture.

However, homeopathic remedies work because they relate to the symptoms, and the person, not because they are "magic pills." The body often takes a long time to recover balance, depending, of course, on the duration of illness. Remedies assist in accelerating the healing and balancing process, but not overnight. They work for the simple reason that they elevate the body to exert its fullest potential in recovery. But potential is rarely reached in a single day. Time and perseverance are part of the underlying principles of homeopathy, especially considering the time it takes to reach imbalance.

Combination remedies have a clear advantage over antacids, aspirin or other pain relievers, as they do not have side effects and can be just as potent. If the intent is to just get better for the moment, without considering the long term, then formula remedies are useful and relatively inexpensive. On the other hand, should your interest in healing be more permanent in nature, then the desired effects must consider deeper, single remedies.

Most of us take pills, whether they are medications, herbs or homeopathic remedies, to recover our health and eliminate the return of symptoms. Ragweed is more a trigger for allergic reactions than it is the actual cause. The specific cause can relate more to an oversensitive adrenal system, overuse of chemicals, inherited tendencies, processed foods, vaccinations or even pollution from the environment.

When we just treat allergic reactions, we do not alter the cause or replenish the adrenal system. We have a temporary resolution, and for some that is all that is needed. For others, elimination on a permanent basis is the ultimate desire. We are a nation desirous of the "quick fix," without consideration for the ill effects that such a "fix" has on the body.

Remember, use combinations for the short term and a single remedy for the long term or chronic illness. For help with the choice of single remedies, consult with a homeopath. Fortunately, homeopathic education has increased over the past decade and there are some excellent practitioners available in North America. Many are non-doctors who specialize in this growing field, which allows the costs to remain reasonable.

In 1990, there were over 37 million people who used alternative medical practices, and combination remedies were considered some of the safest and most reliable ones available. Traditional medicine does not effectively treat certain illnesses, or if it does, side effects are frequently greater than the disease.

A good example is the overuse of antibiotics for children with ear infections. After the antibiotic, the body's natural ability to combat bacteria is diminished and infections keep coming back. Combination remedies eliminate this type of recurrence and assist the body in preventing susceptibility to future disharmonies.

HOW TO USE HOMEOPATHIC REMEDIES

Homeopathic remedies in pill form look and taste like little sugar pills. They also come suspended in alcohol or other type of liquid dilution. When you take the pills, it is best not to touch them with your hands. Most homeopathic remedy containers provide a bottle cap or other type of top to make it easy for you to avoid touching the pills. Just pour the pills out into the top and then directly into your mouth. The pills should be dissolved in the mouth rather than chewed or swallowed.

The liquid remedies can be dropped right on the tongue (don't touch the dropper to your mouth) or added to clean water.

The container will suggest the dose. Dosage is not as important in homeopathy as getting the right remedy. When you are self-treating, it is probably best to use potencies of 6-30x or 6-30c.

Most homeopaths recommend that you not eat or drink anything within 20 or 30 minutes of taking a homeopathic remedy. While you are taking a homeopathic remedy, you should not drink coffee or consume anything containing a strong essential oil such as eucalyptus, tea tree oil or peppermint, menthol and camphor. Other things that can "antidote" or cancel out the effectiveness of homeopathic remedies are drugs, nail polish, and any type of strong negative emotional stress. People respond very differently to homeopathic medicines: some are very sensitive to them and may have them canceled out by relatively minor tastes, smells or events, and in others the remedies keep on working almost regardless of what they do. I recommend you keep a diary of what you notice and how you're feeling.

Homeopathic combinations, when used as directed, and with proven remedies, are safe, effective and rarely have any side effects. You can feel confident that this approach, which has been used for over 200 years, effectively stimulates the immune system rather than diminishes it.

Homeopathy, whether used in combination or as a single remedy, assists the body in rediscovering its natural ability to heal itself. Few other approaches to healing can make that same claim.

CHAPTER 3

62 of the Most Commonly Prescribed Homeopathic Remedies

This chapter is a listing of 62 homeopathic remedies and their "symptoms," as described by homeopath David Dancu. They are only a small portion of the 2,800 remedies available, but they will give you a very good sense of what is available, and what types of symptoms to look for in a homeopathic treatment. According to Dancu, some 70 to 80 percent of all disharmonies treated with homeopathy will be well-served by using one of these remedies. Use this as a general guide, and as a way to familiarize yourself with the essence and identity of each remedy.

Studying and understanding homeopathic remedies is a long-term process. Many remedies have similar traits and symptoms, but each has some unique component to set it apart from the others. These are the aspects that give a deeper comprehension of its essence and help establish a better grasp of the whole remedy.

Aconite: worse after cold, wet weather; anxiety and fears; shock; panic attacks; early or sudden onset of illness; restlessness.

Alumina: anxiety from being hurried; dullness; mental slowness; dryness of all membranes; constipation; disorientation; dizziness; itchiness of the skin without eruptions.

Anacardium: low self-esteem; abusive; cursing; depression; fears and delusions; controlling; violent and angry; brain fatigue; most symptoms are better from eating; strong sexual desires.

Apis: redness, itching, swelling; busy; thirstless; right-sided ailments; worse from heat applications.

Argentum Nitricum: anxiety and panic attacks; impulsive; feelings of abandonment; open and excitable; warm blooded; worse eating sweets, but craves them; gastrointestinal problems; left sided ailments; many phobias.

Arnica: trauma and injuries; concussions; bruises; irritability; prefers to be alone; relief of pains; refuses doctor's help.

Arsenicum Album: anxiety; restlessness; avarice; compulsive; fearful; depressed; skin disharmonies; chilly; controlling without spontaneity; right-sided ailments; worse around midnight; asthma; thirst for small sips; burning sensations.

Aurum: severe suicidal depression; serious; self-condemnation; guilt and abandonment issues; worse cloudy weather; intense; worse with pain; anger with remorse; moans during sleep.

Baryta Carbonica: slowness in mental development; immature behavior; low self-esteem; shy and yielding; anxious and nervous; chronic tonsillitis; blank facial expression.

Belladonna: early onset with redness, heat, flushing of the face and fever; delirium; anger intense with hitting, biting; migraines; thirstless; strep and sore throats.

Bryonia: worse with any movement/motion; irritability; prefers solitude; fear of business or financial failure; dry mucus membranes and dry colon; intense thirst; warm blooded; joint problems.

Calcarea Carbonica: overly responsible; bone problems; fear of heights; fear of going insane; overwhelmed; slow development as a child; stubborn; overweight; slow metabolism; head sweats; milk allergy.

Calcarea Phosphorica: complains about everything; loves change and travel; dissatisfied; sensitive; craves smoked foods; state of weakness; grief with sighing; slow development.

Cantharis: urinary tract infections; burning sensations; strong sexual desires; incontinence; violent emotions.

Carbo Vegetabilise: intense irritability; gastrointestinal problems; negative; prostration and weakness; coma; indifference; coldness; air hunger.

Carcinosin: intense, sympathetic, passionate; family history of cancer; fastidious; craves chocolate and spicy food; moles on back; strong libido; loves animals; low energy from 3 to 6 p.m.; loves travel.

Causticum: idealistic and rebellious; sympathetic; serious; very sensitive to suffering of others; grief;

joint and TMJ problems; warts; compulsive; desires smoked foods; chilly; incontinence.

Chamomilla: peevish when ill; intense irritability; excessive sensitivity to pains; infant desires to be carried; one cheek red, other pale; colic; ear infections; teething problems; worse with travel.

China Officinalis: internal sensitivity; introverted; taciturn; gastrointestinal disharmonies; worse loss of fluids; anemia; colitis; worse touch; periodicity of complaints; fear of animals.

Conium: emotional flatness or indifference; paralysis; cancer; hardness of glands; tumors; fixed ideas; fogginess of the brain.

Cuprum: spasms and convulsions; appears emotionally closed; sensation of suffocating; flat facial expression; seizures; rigid; intense emotions suppressed.

Ferrum Metallicum: anemia; desires raw meat; overweight; face flushes easily; very sensitive to noise; strong willed; better walking slowly; general weakness and fatigue; demanding.

Gelsemium: fatigue; heaviness of the eyelids; brain fatigue; stage fright; weakness of will; cowardly; indifference; forgetful; tremble with anticipation; depressed; thirstless; chilly; headaches; diarrhea.

Graphites: slowness with poor concentration; skin abnormalities; irritable; anxious; herpes; indecisive; many self-doubts; fastidious; overweight tendencies; offensive sweats; restlessness; photophobia.

Hepar Sulphuris: anger when security is threatened; irritable; worse any draft of air; sensitive; chilly; infections and abscesses; intense and hurried; rarely cheerful; abusive; overreacts to pains.

Hyoscyamus: paranoia; jealous with violent outbursts; intense sexual desires; worse with touch; hyperactive child; shameless; defiant; delusions; talkative; fear of dogs; wild gestures.

Ignacia: acute grief or worse since grief; romantic/idealistic; aggravation from consolation; prefers to be alone; stress is better after eating; better with exercise; sighing; disappointed love.

Iodum: very warm; thyroid dysfunctions; very restless and busy; compulsive; talkative and anxious; impulsive; intense appetite; anger; avoids company; discontent and destruction; general fears.

Kali Bichromicum: sinus disharmonies/headaches; strong sense of right and wrong; thick, yellow, ropy discharges; rigid and proper; self-occupied; suppresses emotional aspects of personality.

Kali Carbonicum: righteousness and strong sense of duty; mind rules emotions; fear of losing control; rigid; asthma; possessive; conservative; quarrelsome; self-reproach; worse 2 to 5 a.m.

Lachesis: left-sided complaints; loquacity; suspicious; jealous; sarcastic; opinionated and can be fanatical; warm blooded; all types of menstrual disharmonies; intense personality; vindictive; active mind; drug and alcohol addictions; low self-esteem.

Ledum: prefers solitude; hatred for self and others; joint problems; worse heat, although chilly;

worse movement or motion; irritable; insect bites, lockjaw, or injuries with bruising; puncture wounds.

Lycopodium: poor self-confidence; anger and irritability; liver and kidney disharmonies; fears and anxieties; hyperactive children; right-sided ailments; low energy 4 to 8 p.m.; anticipatory anxiety; tendency to dominate or control; opinionated; avoids responsibility; digestive problems; generally chilly but prefers open air and worse warmth.

Magnesia Muriatica: yielding; aversion to confrontations; feels anxious at night; very responsible; noises annoy; composed, with suppressed inner anger; depression; unrefreshing sleep.

Medorrhinum: nasal discharges; cruel and aggressive behavior; an extremist; "sex, drugs, and rock 'n' roll;" self-centered and loves danger; obsessive/compulsive; history of VD; hurried; intense passions; bites fingernails; overwhelmed by impulses; night person; loves sea.

Mercurius: strong reaction to temperature changes; emotionally closed; stammering speech; conservative; anxious with destructive ideas; paranoia; facade; worse at night; excess saliva; night sweats; serious appearance; metallic taste in mouth; gum infections.

Natrum Carbonicum: very sensitive; craves potatoes; inner turmoil and depression with appearance of cheerfulness; prefers solitude; emotionally closed; sweet and selfless; delicate; poor digestion; worse heat and sun; sadness; milk allergies; sympathetic.

Natrum Muriaticum: fear of being hurt; closed emotionally from past grief; very sensitive; critical; perfectionist; romantic; strong desire for solitude; serious and controlled; introverted; depression; generally worse from being in the sun or heat; hay fever; herpes.

Natrum Sulphuricum: head injuries and concussions; suicidal depressions; very responsible and serious; warm blooded; feels better after a bowel movement; emotionally closed; asthma; possible past history of venereal disease; sensitive; practical, with business focus.

Nitricum Acidum: generally negative person; self-discontent and anger; curses; restless; hypersensitive; selfish; anxieties about health and death; vindictive; chilly pains come and go suddenly.

Nux Vomica: Type "A" personality; ambitious; meticulous; hypersensitive, with tendency to overreact; liver and bowel remedy; driven to excess; addictive personality; sensitive nervous system; intense irritation from wind; chilly; increased hunger.

Petroleum: skin disharmonies of all types, with dryness; quick temper; motion sickness; herpes; offensive perspiration; unable to make decisions; chilly; worse in winter; increased hunger.

Phosphoricum Acidum: dullness and slowness; apathy; feels overwhelmed with grief and emotions; intense fatigue and loss of energy; yielding; desires refreshing fruits; dehydration; chilly.

Phosphorus: expressive and extroverted; prefers consolation and company; impressionable and very sensitive; many fears and anxieties; affectionate; chilly, yet likes cold drinks; craves spicy, salty and sweets; sympathetic; intuitive; nosebleeds.

Platinum: primarily a female remedy; haughty to the extreme; is worse with touch; idealistic; dwells on the past; feels abandoned; dislikes children; insolent and rude; pretentious; strong libido.

Plumbum: taciturn; sad; shy; selfish; difficulty in expressing themselves; indifference; illness slow in development; very chilly; pains tend to radiate; neurological disorders.

Psorinum: skin dysfunction of all types; periodicity; pessimist; tend to despair with hopelessness; anxiety and fear, especially of poverty; very chilly; low energy; feels forsaken/lost; dirty skin.

Pulsatilla: warm-blooded; capricious mood swings; PMS; mild and dependent nature; female remedy; abandonment issues; desires consolation; weepy; digestive and sinus (thick yellow/green mucus) problems; worse heat and craves fresh air; thirstless with dryness.

Rhus Toxicodendron: great internal restlessness; obsessive tendencies; skin and joint remedy; feels better stretching and with motion; withhold affections/feelings; apprehensive at night; timid; herpes with burning and itching; worse cold/damp.

Ruta: affects tendons and fibrous tissues; distrustful; startles easily; argumentative; stiffness/pain; strains; sprains; eyestrain; related headaches; worse motion or lying on painful side.

Sepia: indifference and desire to be alone; impatience; irritability; low sexual desires; chilly; grief and depression; PMS/menopause; bearing down sensations; leucorrhea; taciturn and negative; herpes.

Silica: yielding; timid and bashful; emotionally dependent; low self-esteem; stubborn; chilly; conscientious about details; constipation; slow development; weakness; perspires easily; recurring infections.

Spigelia: left sided ailments; serious; responsible; violent pains; migraines; grief; worse tobacco smoke; anxiety of pointed objects; pinworms; combination heart and eye symptoms; chilly; worse touch.

Spongia: fear of suffocation; heart ailments; increased anxiety; dry mucus membranes; dry, barking, croupy cough; easily frightened; thyroid disharmonies; respiratory conditions; weakness.

Staphysagria: sweet, yielding person; suppressed emotions; very sensitive; emotionally dependent; fear of losing control; possible history of sexual abuse or humiliation; strong sexual history; grief; suppressed anger; low self-confidence; worse after nap; mild.

Stramonium: violent tendencies; etiology from a fright; impulsive rage; wild behavior; night terror; desires company and light; intense thirst; flushed face; excitable; stammers; convulsions; promiscuous; hyperactive children; could be mild, gentle and very sensitive.

Sulphur: idealistic and philosophical; self-contained; indolent; warm blooded; burning sensations; desires spicy foods; appearance is not important; collect things; opinionated; desires open air; itch; offensive discharges; offended by others' body odor; aversion to bathing.

Syphilinum: compulsive tendencies; worse at night; very chilly; alcoholic; excess saliva; fear of disease/germs or going insane; nails are distorted; anxious; indifferent; worse hot or cold extremes.

Thuja: low self-confidence; emotionally closed and hard to get to know; secretive; fastidious; hurried; herpes and suppressed venereal disease; ailments after vaccinations; urine stream is forked; runny nose with stool; chilly; left sided ailments; irritable; warts; oily skin.

Tuberculinum: desires change and travel; feels unfulfilled; can be mean; compulsive; chilly; respiratory disharmonies; milk and cat allergies; hyperactive children; romantic longings; desires smoked foods; excess perspiration at night; itch, better with heat.

Veratrum Album: self-righteous and haughty; thinking more than feeling; precocious child; hyperactive child; ambitious; deceitful; very chilly; abusive spouse; critical; jealous; restlessness; religious mania; excessive cold sweats; inappropriate kissing or hugging.

Zincum: hypersensitive and overstimulated; impulsive movements; restlessness; always complaining; mentally overwhelmed and fatigued; worse when drinking wine or alcohol; superstitious; chilly; affected by noises; feels better after eating.

CHAPTER 4

Remedies for Short-Term, Acute Illnesses

Homeopathic self-treatment and combination remedies are best suited to acute illnesses. An acute illness is self-limiting, meaning that it has a life span of approximately seven to ten days. Without any treatment, it usually goes away on its own. The following chapter is a compilation of the most common acute remedies as compiled by homeopath, teacher and author David Dancu.

Homeopathy is not used for every symptom that arises, as these symptoms are the body's messages of disharmony. A fever is a message that there is an infection and body heat is a means of disarming or eliminating the infection. By allowing the body to function as much as possible without outside influences, it finds a way to recover and regain its energy, balance and strength.

The following list of remedies covers a variety of acute illnesses along with some proven remedies. These brief symptoms will help you in using homeopathy for short-term acute illnesses and can be helpful in some emergencies. Obviously, if there is a crisis or critical situation, common sense dictates that proper medical treatment be obtained. On the other hand, homeopathic remedies are excellent for shock and emergencies while a person is being transported to the hospital or health care provider.

ACCIDENTS

Abrasions/cuts

Arnica for trauma of all types and bleeding, even coma.
Calendula for antiseptic use, either internal or external.
Hypericum for injury to nerve endings or incisions.
Ledum helps heal puncture and penetration wounds.

Burns

Cantharis reduces pain and promotes healing process.
Urtica Urens for first- and second-degree burns.
Hypericum reduces pain when nerve endings are involved such as spine, fingers and teeth.
Belladonna for fever, flushing of the face and delirium.

Bites

Ledum for all types of bites with coldness around area.
Hypericum when pain seems excessive for the wound.
Belladonna for dog and snake bites.
Lachesis for snake bites or with flushes of heat.

Bruises

Arnica for bruises or muscle injuries.
Bellis for trauma, contusions and soreness.
Hamamelis helps with internal bleeding and bruising.
Ruta for stiffness in muscles and tendons from bruising.

Bleeding

Phosphorus for all types of hemorrhaging.
Ferrum Phosphoricum helps coagulate the blood.
Lachesis when blood is dark and area is blue.
Ipecacuanha for gushing, bright red blood with nausea.

Head Injuries

Arnica for all types; conscious or unconscious.
Cicuta for dilated pupils, muscle spasms and stiffness.
Gelsemium for occipital pain and heaviness of the eyes.
Hypericum for numbness, tingling and seizures.

Shock

Aconite after sudden fright or fearful situation.
Arnica after an injury or trauma, causing shock.
Carbo Vegetabilis for fainting, coldness and difficulty breathing.
Veratrum Album when skin and perspiration are very cold.

Whiplash

Bryonia when any movement is painful.
Causticum when neck muscles and tendons contract.
Hypericum if nerves and a tingling sensation are involved.
Rhus Tox for injuries that are better with motion and heat.

ALLERGIES

Anaphylactic Shock

Apis for constriction, inflammation, swelling, hives, redness of the skin and soreness; worse with heat.
Urtica Urens for eruptions, itching, blotches and burning; heat with a stinging sensation.
Consider: Arsenicum Album; Natrum Mur; Rhus Tox.

To Animals

Arsenicum Album for respiratory-related reactions.
Allium Cepa for clear, burning nasal discharge with runny eyes.
Euphrasia for profuse, burning discharge from eyes.
Natrum Mur for egg white-like discharge; cannot smell.
Consider: Sabadilla, Nux Vomica; Tuberculinum; Sulphur.

To Chemicals

Arsenicum when there is a burning sensation after exposure.

Coffea for excitability of the mind and nervousness.

Mercurius when you feel worse at night with excess sweat.

Nitricum Acid for the oversensitive, depressed and negative types.

Consider: Nux Vomica, Phosphorus; Sulphur; Psorinum.

To Dust

Arsenicum Album when respiration/wheezing is involved.

Bromium when there is a feeling of suffocation and coldness.

Hepar for heart palpitations and anxious wheezing.

Consider: Silica; Ipecacuanha; Pothos.

To Foods

Beans: Bryonia; Lycocpodium; Petroleum; Calcarea Carb.

Bread: Bryonia; Lycopodium; Natrum Mur; Pulsatilla; Sepia.

Cheese: Arsenicum; Nux Vomica; Phosphorus; Sepia.

Coffee: Cantharis; Causticum; Chamomilla; Nux Vomica.

Fruit: Arsenicum; Bryonia; China; Colocynthis; Pulsatilla.

Meat: Arsenicum; Calcarea; China; Ferrum; Kali Carb.

Milk: Calcarea; China; Magnesium Mur; Natrum Carb; Sepia.

Onions: Lycopodium; Thuja; Sulphur; Ignacia; Pulsatilla.

Potatoes: Aluminum; Bryonia; Silica; Sepia; Pulsatilla.

Salt: Carbo Vegetabilis; Natrum Mur; Drosera; Phosphorus; Silica.

Starches: Berberis; Lycopodium; Natrum Mur; Lachesis.

Sugar: Argentum Nit; Lycopodium; Sulphur; Phosphorus.

Vegetables: Aluminum; Bryonia; Kali Carb; Natrum Sulph.

Wheat: Allium cepa; Lycopodium; Natrum Mur; Pulsatilla.

Hay Fever

Arsenicum Iod. for profuse watery discharges and tickling.

Wyethia for itching of the palate and dry mucous membranes.

Arundo for burning and itch in nostrils with sneezing.

Arum for sneezing and tickling sensations; congestion.

Consider: Arsenicum; Allium Cepa; Sabadilla; Euphrasia.

Insect Bites

Ledum for any puncture wound with coldness around the wound.

Apis for red, hot, swollen skin that is worse with heat.

Hypericum for tingling sensations or numbness.
Urtica Urens for hives, itching, redness and worse with heat.
Consider: Arsenicum; Belladonna; Thuja; Lachesis.

Poison Ivy

Bryonia has swelling, heat, dryness, thirst and is irritable.
Anacardium for intense itch with swelling and redness.
Croton Tig. for painful scratching and pustules; intense.
Graphites for a watery discharge from the reaction.
Consider: Clematis; Rhus Tox; Sepia; Sanguianaria.

To Smoke

Euphrasia for burning in the eyes and nasal discharge.
Ignacia when breathing is affected; person feels annoyed.
Sepia for nausea and exhaustion with any left-sidedness.
Spigelia for dryness, tickling and constriction in throat.
Consider: Nux Vomica; Natrum Mur; Causticum; Sulphur.

CHILDREN'S REMEDIES

Colic

Chamomilla desires to be carried, is irritable and angry.

Colocynthis for a bloated stomach with intense pains.
Dioscorea for arching back with cramping pains and gas.
Magnesia Phos when a child feels better bending double with the cramps.

Chicken Pox

Aconite for the first stages of the outbreak.
Antimonium Crudum when overheated and angry.
Rhus Tox for restless, intense itch with swollen glands.
Sulphur for a burning itch which is worse in heat and sweat.

Colds

Aconite for sudden onset from cold, dry winds.
Belladonna for early stage with fever, redness and thirst.
Kali Bic when discharge is thick yellow/green and ropy.
Pulsatilla for thick yellow mucus and clinging to parent.
Consider: Allium Cepa; Euphrasia; Hepar; Nux Vomica.

Coughs

Barking: Aconite; Belladonna; Drosera; Spongia.
Croupy: Aconite; Hepar Sulphuris; Spongia; Lachesis; Phos.
Dry: Belladonna; Bryonia; Drosera; Natrum Mur; Rumex.

Hacking: Allium Cepa; Arsenicum; Drosera; Phosphorus.

Rattling: Antimonium Tart; Causticum; Dulcamura; Ipecacuanha.

Violent: Belladonna; Causticum; Cuprum; Lachesis; Phosphorus.

Whooping: Antimonium Tart; Carbo Vegetabilis; Cuprum; Drosera.

Diarrhea

Arsenicum for a watery, burning stool with nausea.

China for a painless stool containing undigested food.

Podophyllum for a frequent, gushing stool that is smelly.

Rheum for sour smelling stool resulting from teething.

Consider: Nux Vomica, Sulphur; Silica; Rhus Tox.

Earache

Aconite for the early stages with cold symptoms.

Chamomilla when pain and irritability arise together.

Hepar for smelly discharges; is worse when cold.

Pulsatilla for congestion with redness and discharge.

Consider: Lycopodium; Silica; Mercurius; Belladonna.

Fevers

Aconite for sudden onset with anxiety, heat and dryness.

Belladonna for flushed face, burning heat and delirium.

Gelsemium for shivering, heat, drowsiness and no sweat.

Mercurius for excess saliva; heat alternates with chills.

Consider: Natrum Mur; Nux Vomica; Pulsatilla; Sulphur.

Influenza

Oscillococcinum for the earliest stages, within 24 hours.

Baptisia for prostration, muscle soreness and stomach.

Eupatorium when there is deep bone ache and debility.

Gelsemium for drowsiness, aches, chills and exhaustion.

Consider: Arsenicum; Bryonia; Rhus Tox; Nux Vomica.

Indigestion

China when gas arises after eating fruit; bloated.

Ignacia when problem is caused by any type of emotional upset.

Lycopodium for gas and bloating made worse by eating.

Nux Vomica from overindulgence of food or drink.

Consider: Argentum. Nitninme; Pulsatilla; Carbo Vegetabilis; Sulphur.

Measles

Aconite is excellent for early stages.
Belladonna for fever; is used in the early stages.
Bryonia for cough, fever, dryness and intense thirst.
Pulsatilla is restless and desires attention; no thirst.
Consider: Gelsemium; Apis; Euphrasia; Phosphorus.

Mumps

Belladonna for swelling, fever, heat and redness.
Jaborandi for redness, swollen glands and excess saliva.
Mercurius for painful swelling, fever and profuse sweat.
Rhus Tox for swelling with fever; better with heat.
Consider: Aconite, Apis; Lachesis; Phytolacca; Pulsatilla.

Rash (Diaper)

Apis for red, sore, shiny and hot skin; worse with heat.
Petroleum for dry, red, itching and cracked skin.
Rhus Tox when it is better with hot baths; skin itches, flakes and burns.
Sulphuricum Acidum for blotchy, red skin; worse with heat.
Consider: Sulphur; Graphites; Mezereum; Urtica Urens.

Sore Throat

Aconite for heat and fever from dry cold winds.
Belladonna is the first choice with heat and redness.
Causticum for burning, soreness, rawness and tightness.
Phytolacca for congestion, redness and very painful.
Consider: Apis; Hepar; Lachesis; Mercurius; Gelsemium.

Teething

Belladonna for pain, fever, shrieking, restless and flushed.
Calcarea Phos for slow, difficult dentition.
Chamomilla for intense pain, irritability and hot cheeks.
Pulsatilla for clinginess; painful dentition. Better in fresh air.
Consider: Coffea; Silica; Kreosotum; Rheum; Phytolacca.

HEADACHES

Migraine:

Bryonia for a pressing sensation with thirst; worse with motion.
Gelsemium for dull, droopy mind fog; blurred vision.
Glonoinium for throbbing pain, heaviness and irritability.

Melilotus for bursting pain with red face and nausea.

Sanguinaria for right-sided pain that radiates to eye; worse in the a.m.

Consider: Belladonna; Iris; Coffea; Apis; Nux Vomica; Spigelia.

Tension

Argentum Nitricum for an enlarged head feeling with impulsiveness.

Ignacia when you feel worse from any emotional stress or anxiety.

Natrum Mur feels like pounding hammers; worse 10:00 a.m.; throbs.

Phosphoric Acid when apathetic; worse from loss of fluids or emotions.

Zincum when exhausted, nervous and restless; noise sensitive.

Consider: Coffea; Gelsemium; China; Nux Vomica; Thuja; Phos.

Hormonal

Cyclamen for a flickering sensation; worse in open air and when chilled.

Kreosotum for menstrual headaches with irritability.

Lachesis for deep pain, coming in waves; left-sided with burning.

Sepia feels as if there is a band around the head; left side; sad.

Pulsatilla for when you feel weepy, sad, thirstless and are sweating; better in open air.

Consider: Lycopodium; Natrum Mur; Belladonna; Lac Caninum.

Sick

Cocculus for motion sickness, loss of sleep or noise.

Chelidonium for liver-related and right-sided sickness with drowsiness.

Nux Vomica for overindulgence of any kind.

Picric Acid for mental strain, fatigue or travel.

Consider: Iris; Ipecacuanha; Sulphur; Arsenicum Album; Sanguinaria.

Sinus

Dulcamara for changes in barometric pressure; worse in damp air.

Euphrasia for burning sensation in the eyes with tearing.

Kali Bic for burning sensation at root of nose; pain in one area; sinusitis.

Mercurius for excess saliva, bad breath and metallic taste.

Consider: Calcarea Sulph; Hepar; Nux Vomica; Thuja; Natrum Mur.

Periodic

Arsenicum for one specific time of day with burning; better with heat.

China when worse from loss of fluids or malaria; liver ailments.

Nitricum Acidum for burning nasal discharge; worse with pressure.

Silica for radiating pains, head sweats, worse drafts, chills.

Consider: Natrum Mur; Sanguinaria; Sepia; Lachesis; Ignacia.

SPORTS INJURIES

Broken Bones/Fractures

Arnica for the earliest stage of trauma or injury.
Bryonia when pain is intense from any type of motion.
Calcarea Phos helps in formation of callus in fractures.
Symphytum helps bones to properly knit after being set.
Consider: Hypericum; Rhus Tox; Ruta; Silica; Calcarea.

Dislocations

Carbo Animalis for diminished strength and tendon contraction.
Kali Nitricum for numbness, heaviness and weakness of limbs.
Calcarea when the problem is chronic and fails to heal.
Ruta when tendons are involved, especially wrist and ankle.
Consider: Arnica; Natrum Carb; Rhus Tox; Lycopodium; Bryonia.

Pulled Hamstring

Bellis for soreness, stiffness, coldness and bruising.

Ambra-G for drawing pain; limb seems shortened; tingling.

Causticum for hardness of tendons and contractions; cramps.

Ledum for swelling and stiffness; better with ice.

Consider: Arnica; Ruta; Rhus Tox; Bryonia; Sulphuricum Acidum.

Hip Pointers

Aesculus for radiating pain that is worse upon standing.

Calcarea Phos for stiffness; worse with motion or air drafts.

Rhus Tox if stretching reduces pain; better with heat.

Ruta for lameness and stiffness; better when lying down.

Consider: Arnica; Bellis; Hamamelis; Symphytum; Bryonia.

Sprains/Strains

Bryonia when worse from any movement; wants to be alone.

Bellis for stiffness with a bruised sensation.

Asafoetida for hysteria with bone pains and inflammation.

Millefolium for tearing pains from overexertion; irritable.

Consider: Arnica (first); Rhus Tox; Ruta; Ledum.

TRAVEL

Constipation

Alumina when patient has no desire for stool or may strain; straining; worse with travel.

Bryonia for dark, dry, hard stool; very thirsty for cold water.

Nux Vomica when bloated and irritable; never feels fully vacated.

Silica for ineffectual urging; hard stool which pulls back in.

Consider: Plumbum; Sulphur; Opium; Aloe; Sepia; Nitricum Acidum.

Diarrhea

Aconite after cold, dry wind or fright.

Arsenicum for prostration, vomiting, restlessness and anxiety.

China after eating fruit or a summer chill; painless; fever.

Colocynthis for intense colicky pains; better with pressure.

Consider: Nux Vomica; Veratrum Album; Podophyllum; Aloe; Sulphur.

Indigestion

Anacardium for heartburn two hours after eating; pain/fullness.

Carbo Vegetabilis for offensive gas, bloating, pain and internal heat.

Lycopodium when bloated with pain; better after passing gas.

Nux Vomica when worse after overeating; gas, bloating and cramping.

Consider: Arsenicum; Bryonia; China; Pulsatilla; Sulphur; Hepar.

Influenza/Cold

Ferrum Phos for the earliest stages without clear symptoms.

Baptisia for prostration, cramps, nausea and confusion.

Gelsemium when achy, chilled, weak and anxious; heavy eyelids.

Eupatorium Perf. for deep bone aches with chills and headache.

Consider: Arsenicum; Bryonia; Nux Vomica; Rhus Tox; Hepar.

Jet Lag

Cocculus when lack of sleep causes irritability and fatigue.

Gelsemium for heavy eyes, headache, weakness and tired limbs.

Argentum Nitricum for fear and panic while flying; anxious.

Arnica for being cramped in a seat for a long period.

Consider: Rescue Remedy; Phos Acid; Zincum; Sulphuricum Acidum.

Motion Sickness

Borax for nausea or vomiting; worse with downward motion.

Cocculus for queasiness; worse with the thought of food.

Nux Vomica for nausea, headache and chills; no desire for food.

Tabacum when chilled, giddy and sweating; worse with tobacco smoke.
Consider: Rhus Tox; Petroleum; Ipecacuanha.

Sleeplessness

Arsenicum for restlessness, anxiety, fatigue and irritability.
Coffea when nervous, anxious, hypersensitive and mentally active.
Ignacia when worse from emotional stress or grief.
Nux Vomica when worse from overeating, alcohol or mental strain.
Consider: Aconite; Lycopodium; Pulsatilla; Arnica.

Stress

Natrum Mur for long-term emotional ill effects and solitude.
Nux Vomica when there is mental stress and overstimulation.
Passiflora when overworked, worried, restless and exhausted.
Valerian when oversensitive, irritable, nervous and changeable.
Consider: Zincum; Arsenicum; Argent Nit; Ignacia; Sepia.

WOMEN'S AILMENTS

Cystitis

Apis for burning, stinging and soreness when urinating.
Cantharis for intense urging, burning which is passed by drops.

Equisetum for bladder fullness, severe pain and frequent urge.

Lycopodium for low back pains, straining and retention.

Consider: Aconite; Belladonna; Lachesis; Sepia; Pulsatilla.

Discharges

Black: China; Kreosotum; Rhus Tox; Secale.

Bloody: Calcarea Sulph; China; Cocculus; Nitricum Acidum; Sepia.

Burning: Calcarea; Borax; Kreosotum; Pulsatilla; Sulphur.

Green: Carbo Vegetabilis; Kali Bic; Mercurius; Natrum Mur; Sepia.

Itching: Calcarea; China; Mercurius; Sepia; Kreosotum; Zincum.

Milky: Calcarea; Kali Mur; Sepia; Silica; Pulsatilla; Lachesis.

Offensive: Kali Arsenicum; Kreosotum; Mercurius; Nux Vomica.

Profuse: Calcarea; Graphites; Sepia; Silica; Stannum; Thuja.

Thick: Arsenicum; Calcarea; Kali Bic; Natrum Carb; Thuja; Zinc

Thin: Graphites; Nitricum Acidum; Pulsatilla; Sulphur; Silica; Sepia.

White: Borax; Graphites; Natrum Mur; Sepia; Nux Vomica; Pulsatilla.

Yellow: Arsenicum; Calcarea; Chamomilla; Hydrastis; Pulsatilla.

Genital Herpes

Natrum Mur for tingling sensations; worse in sun or under stress.

Petroleum for sensations of moisture with crusting and itch.

Sepia for itching, worse at folds of skin and in spring; odor.

Thuja for eruptions on covered parts only; sensitive to touch.

Consider: Rhus Tox; Alnus; Medorrhinum; Lachesis; Dulcamura.

Menopause

Lachesis for hot flashes and fainting; worse with tight clothing.

Lilium Tig for intensity, depression, irritability and prolapsed.

Pulsatilla when clingy, complaining, weepy and sad; worse with heat.

Sepia when overwhelmed and irritable; prefers solitude; hot flashes.

Consider: Sulphur; Natrum Mur; Phosphorus; Sabina; Kreosotum.

Menses

Absent: Aurum; Ferrum; Graphites; Kali Carb; Lycopodium; Pulsatilla.

Clotted: Belladonna; Calcarea; China; Lachesis; Sabina; Pulsatilla.

Cramps: Chamomilla; Cocculus; Colocynthis; Mag Phos; Sepia.

Frequent: Arsenicum; Belladonna; Cyclamen; Ferrum Phos.

Irregular: Argent Nit; Nux Moschata; Pulsatilla; Sepia; Senecio.

Late: Causticum; Cuprum; Lachesis; Natrum Mur; Sarsaparilla.

Painful: Cimicifuga; Mag Phos; Millefolium; Cactus; Pulsatilla; Sabina; Sulphur; Caulophyllum; Cyclamen; Chamomilla.
Profuse: Arsenicum; Ferrum Phos; Phos; Calcarea Phos; Sabina; Senecio; Millefolium; Natrum Mur; Ferrum; Cyclamen.
Suppressed: Belladonna; Cyclamen; Lachesis; Senecio; Sepia.

Pelvic Inflammatory Disease

Arsenicum for burning, offensive discharge with anxiety.
Lac Caninum for ovarian pains and vaginal gas; fear of snakes.
Lachesis for left-sided pains and cysts; worse with tight clothing.
Sabina for severe PMS, intense pains, gushing flow; leucorrhea.
Consider: Apis; Belladonna; Cantharis; Pulsatilla; Chamomilla; Sepia.

Vaginitis

Medorrhinum for high sex drive and chronic infection; herpes.
Pulsatilla when needy and capricious; does not tolerate pain.
Thuja for green discharges, herpes, polyps and cysts.
Kreosotum for strong itch with burning discharge and odor.
Consider: Arsenicum; Graphites; Mercurius; Sepia; Sulphur.

CHAPTER 5

The Homeopathic First Aid Kit

Many homeopathic remedies are useful as immediate treatment in the case of injury or accident. Homeopathic treatment for emergencies does not require the detailed taking of a case needed for chronic illnesses. Only a small number of remedies apply. It is important to remember that homeopathic medicines should not be used in place of standard first aid measures. Always perform these procedures first and summon help when needed.

For on-the-spot treatment, besides pellets and tablets, homeopathic tinctures can be applied directly to injured sites. Tinctures are prepared with alcohol which can sting cuts and broken skin.

It's always worth using topical applications made from the original substances of certain homeopathic remedies such as calendula. The creams and lotions make very effective support for remedies taken internally.

FIRST AID DOSES

Common dosage of homeopathic remedies in first aid is two tablets, three to four times a day. This can increase to two tablets every 30 minutes to one hour when pain is severe. Reduce the frequency as improvement begins, but continue dosing until improvement is well established.

Remedy	Used for	Benefits
Arnica (Internal and as oil or ointment. Use before other remedies to treat the shock of any injury.)	Bleeding under skin Bruises, ordinary Burns (Treatment for shock only) Fractures Injuries from blows or falls Bee, hornet and wasp stings Jagged cuts (internal remedy only) Muscular soreness Shin splints Shock Soreness, general Strains, general Strained back muscles Twisted knee (Take on first day)	Speeds healing. Relieves pain. Reduces swelling.
Bryonia	Injured joint (swollen, distended, worse with movement) Twisted knee (take on 2nd day if worse with movement) Fractured ribs	Relieves pain. Speeds healing.
Calendula (Nonalcoholic lotion for cuts or ointment for scrapes,	Abrasions Bee, hornet and wasp stings Bleeding from mouth Burns, 1st degree (add	Cleanses and speeds healing of slight wounds. Helps stop

etc. Saturate dressing with lotion. (Lotion or ointment)	drops to cold water treatment.) Jock itch Scratches Superficial wounds	bleeding. Inhibits infection.
Cantharis	Burns, 3rd degree (internally only)	Speeds healing.
Glonoinium	Sunstroke and heat exhaustion	Speeds recovery.
Hypericum (Lotion for external use)	Crushed nerves Burns, 2nd degree (Immerse in lotion) Nerve injuries to extremities and elbows Puncture wounds	Promotes tissue growth. Speeds healing. Relieves pain.
Ledum (Lotion for external use)	Bee, hornet, wasp stings Bruises (cold, numb, long-lasting) Black eye Puncture wounds Splinter under nail Swelling	Reduces pain and inflammation, especially when wound relieved by cold.
Rhus Toxicodendron (Use after Arnica)	Blistery itches Injury after lifting/overexertion Joints, creaky Joints, hot, swollen Strained/torn muscles, tendons, ligaments Poison Ivy/Oak Tendonitis	Relieves aches and itching. Speeds healing.

Ruta
(Use after
Arnica and
when Rhus
Tox has not
helped)

Bruised bone covering
Injuries to bones
Lame feeling
Prolapsed, protruding
rectum
Soft tissue injuries
Sprains to ankle/wrist
Strained/torn muscles
(when initial swelling
has decreased)

Speeds
healing.

RESOURCES AND REFERENCES

David A. Dancu, N.D. is a practicing homeopath who teaches and has a private practice in Boulder, Colorado. His new book, *Homeopathic Vibrations . . . A Guide for Natural Healing* (Sunshine Press, 1996) is available through book stores or by mail for $22.95 (P.O. Box 333, Hygiene, CO 80533).

Bellavite, P., Signorini, A., *Homeopathy, A Frontier in Medical Science*, North Atlantic Books, Calif., 1995.

Boericke & Tafel, *The Family Guide to Self-medication, Homeopathic*, Boericke & Tafel, Inc., Calif. 1988.

Cummings, S., Ullman, D., *Everybody's Guide to Homeopathic Medicines*, G.P. Putnam's Sons, New York, 1991.

Dancu, D.A., *Homeopathic Vibrations, A Guide to Natural Healing*, Sunshine Press, Boulder, Colo., 1996.

Hamilton, S., "What You Should Know About Homeopathy," *American Health*, December 1995.

Kahn, J., "Homeopathic Remedy Relieves Allergic Asthma Symptoms," *Medical Tribune*, 11, January 5, 1995.

Panos, M. B., Heimlich, J., *Homeopathic Medicine at Home*, G.P. Putnam's Sons, New York., 1980.

Reilly, D. et al, "Is Evidence for Homeopathy Reproducible?" *The Lancet*, 344:1601-1606, December 10, 1994.

"Homeopathy Scores Again," *Townsend Letter for Doctors & Patients*, p.27, June 1996.

Ullman, D., *The Consumer's Guide to Homeopathy*, G.P. Putnam's Sons, New York, 1995.

Hill, N., et al, "A Placebo Controlled Clinical Trial Investigating the Efficacy of a Homeopathic After-Bite Gel in Reducing Mosquito Bite Induced Erythema," *European Journal of Clinical Pharmacology*, 49:103-108, 1995.

INDEX

Dr. Earl Mindell's

What You Should Know About . . .
series
in print or forthcoming